Breathing Better

—

Feeling Better

Breathing Better

—

Feeling Better

*A guide to Feeling Better by
Breathing Better*

Cecile Cates Gegg

To order additional copies of this book, contact:
Xlibris Corporation
1-888-795-4274
www.Xlibris.com
Orders@Xlibris.com
84238

To Elyse, Shane, Joey, Charly and Jaime.

CONTENTS

CHAPTER ONE

BENEFITS OF BREATHING PROPERLY

Because oxygen is vital to these bodies we inhabit, learning how to breathe properly is essential to feeling our best. Learning to breathe properly not only feeds our bodies the Life Force that keeps us alive, it also feeds our brains. And, failure to breathe properly decreases our oxygen which results in increased stress, loss of energy, sleeplessness and low mental focus.

One of the first things that people are told when they become excited or agitated is to 'take a deep breath'. This is because there are magic healing qualities in our breath.

When we become fearful, excited, nervous, anxious, or stressed in any way, our breathing becomes more rapid. By simply taking a few deep breaths, we allow our bodies and minds to relax thereby bringing us back into the present moment. How powerful this simple act of taking a few deep breaths!

The way we breathe has the ability to influence our states of mind. How we breathe can calm or excite us, relax or tense us, as well as confuse or clear our minds. Each time we inhale, we bring oxygen into the body which sparks the conversion of nutrients into fuel. And, on each exhalation we rid the body of carbon dioxide (toxic waste). Slow focused mindful breathing allows the body and mind to relax, and as a result one begins to feel a sense of calming stillness. Sadly, there are so many of us who either aren't aware or who choose to ignore the ability that breathing has to affect our bodies, minds and spirits.

We are all searching (whether consciously or unconsciously) for ways to feel better and to be happier. Ultimately it's about developing a sense of peace within ourselves so that we don't have to be constantly doing, talking, buying and moving in order to be happy. Once we find the peace that is our true nature, we won't always have to be doing. Someone said once—we are human beings, not human doings. Learning how to breathe better, finding the rhythm of your breath (Life Force), as it comes in and out of your body, will bring you what you are really looking for—peace. Then from this sense of peace, you will be able to live a fuller, less stressed life, knowing that deep down, under all the craziness of the world, everything is OK, all is well. It is what it is! That acceptance is peace.

Breathwork has been proven to be one of the oldest and most effective ways to reduce stress and improve overall health and well-being. Bringing focus to the breath enables us to clear our minds when our thoughts have run away and we are feeling confused or frustrated. The moment we begin to focus on the breath, our minds begin to relax, because when we focus on our breath coming in and going out, our minds are unable to think of anything else. A perfect breath is when we inhale fully filling the entire diaphragm, and then holding the breath for just a moment before we begin to exhale slowly and completely. The rhythm of our breath is unique to each and every one of us, and only with practice are we able to find that perfect rhythm.

Athletes are taught how important breathing is for maximum results. Swimmers are taught how to breathe with each stroke, and runners are taught how to breathe to maximize stamina. Also, singers and those who play musical instruments requiring breath learn how to breathe in order to produce better sounds. What do these people know that the average person doesn't? They know how important and how powerful their breath can be. So, learning how to breathe more effectively, gives us the ability to control what we might not have realized we had the ability to control.

In addition, we are also able to relieve pain, or at the very least to reduce pain, by focusing on our breathing. Women who are birthing their children without the use of drugs are taught to breathe into each contraction to lessen the discomfort.

By changing our breathing, we have the power to change how we feel at any given moment—mentally, physically and emotionally. Our breath is a gift that most of us aren't using to the fullest in order to live a more peaceful life.

My experience practicing Yoga has taught me how important our breath is—the primary source of energy or Life Force that permeates the entire universe. Every living organism breathes!

The practice of Yoga has increased in the West, and because Yoga focuses extensively on the breath, there are many that have become more aware of the benefits of proper breathing through this practice. Since breathing is one of the eight limbs of Yoga, it's as equally important as the postures that are practiced. However, one doesn't need to actually practice the physical postures of Yoga in order to benefit from breathing properly. We all breathe, every living creature breathes, and what I'm hoping to accomplish in writing this little book is to provide an easy understanding of the importance of proper breathing as well as some useful techniques to practice better breathing.

Even though these breathing techniques are Yoga based, this book is not about Yoga as we in the West have come to think of this increasingly popular practice. The benefits of breathing properly can be experienced by all of us; all we have to do is slow down and begin to focus on the breath . . . . our Life Force. Our breath coming in and going back out is the miracle of our being alive. The first breath is taken when we are born, and the last breath is taken just before we leave. And yet, most of us have never given a second thought to our breath, unless of course we have developed breathing problems or have found ourselves in a situation where there isn't enough air. Each time we inhale, we bring oxygen into the body which sparks the conversion of nutrients into fuel. And, on each exhalation we rid the body of carbon dioxide (toxic waste).

Equally important is how bringing awareness to your breath as it enters and leaves your body, actually allows your mind to relax. Our minds think thousands of thoughts every day, and most of these are the same thoughts we thought yesterday.

Because we live in a very stressful time, the need to find a way to relax, and become more peaceful is increasing, and learning to breathe properly is a simple and quick way to help us find that peace. Most of us are so busy living our lives, we don't think of giving any attention to something as basic as breathing. However, once we recognize that the simple act of breathing has the power to affect our bodies, minds and spirits, we will have the opportunity to relieve some of the stress that is so prevalent at this time.

We all want to feel better. We want to be able to welcome life as it comes, the good and the not so good, to accept and manage the difficulties that we experience in our daily lives, without reacting through anger and/or fear. We've all heard it said that it's not what happens to us, it's how we *feel* about what happens to us. With the practice of these few basic breathing techniques, you will begin to feel more relaxed and peaceful. We all have choices—we can go through life stressed and unhappy, or we can develop ways to accept life without allowing it to overwhelm us, thus reducing stress and illness. Slow focused mindful breathing allows the body and mind to relax, and as a result one begins to feel a sense of calming stillness.

We all deserve to know how important our breath is, and how simple it is to breathe better. Once you have practiced these simple breathing techniques, you'll begin to realize that you have the ability to change the way you feel at any given moment, simply by changing the way that you breathe. Athletes, singers, as well as mothers giving birth, all know the importance of proper focused breathing. Now, we can all learn how to feel better through breathing better.

Inhaling through our nostrils, holding the breath for just a moment, and then exhaling through our nostrils, creating a nice smooth rhythm, is the best and most beneficial way to breathe. We humans all tend to breathe very shallowly, which means that we breathe only into the top portions of our lungs. As a result, this leaves the remainder of our lungs stagnant, and usually filled with stale air. Focusing on our exhalation is very important, as this empties out our lungs in order to make room for a deeper inhalation. We need not worry about inhaling, our bodies will naturally take a breath when they feel threatened there isn't enough air. The key to better breathing is to focus on exhaling—this is where the sense of relaxation begins. It's about letting go—something that is very difficult for many of us. When we focus on exhaling, we are letting go of our breath slowly and mindfully. This allows are minds and our bodies to begin to unwind, resulting in a sense of relaxation and peacefulness.

Ultimately we all want to feel more peaceful. Being peaceful allows us to be in harmony with whatever happens in our lives—accepting life as it comes, one moment at a time. These are stressful times in which we live, just look at how many medications are available on the market geared toward helping people cope better. We all have within us the ability to feel peaceful and relaxed—all we have to do is learn how to breathe better in order to feel better. Once we learn how to relax at will, we no longer have to be at the mercy of outside circumstances that we have previously allowed to stress and upset us. I'm offering you some breathing techniques that you will be able to practice at will. By bringing your awareness to your breath, you are bringing your awareness back into the present moment, the now. You may not be able to change your circumstances, however you most definitely have the ability to change the way you feel about whatever is happening in your life. Change the way you look at things and the things you look at change.

CHAPTER TWO

OUR BREATH IS OUR LIFE FORCE

The breath that comes in and out of our bodies is what keeps us alive. The oxygen in that breath is what feeds our bodies and our brains. Simply put, **Our Breath Is Our Life Force**. Without this breath there is no life.

How we breathe has a definite impact on how we feel. Simply by changing the way we breathe, we can change how we feel physically, mentally and emotionally. Just take a moment and inhale a nice deep breath, and exhale a long complete exhalation . . . . notice how this makes you feel!

Our breath is something that most of us don't even think about. We take our first breath when we enter this world and our last breath when we leave. How many of us can honestly say that we have ever given any thought to whether there would be enough breath for us to breathe, it's something we all take for granted. This is the miracle of being alive, the fact that these bodies breathe . . . . without any effort on our part. It's just something that happens and we take it for granted.

If we were more aware of the importance of this breath, I believe that we would all make a more conscious effort to breathe better. By bringing our awareness to our breath, we can begin to use it to relax us, to rejuvenate us and to simply help us feel better. This ultimately allows us to become more peaceful. Knowing that we have the ability to change how we feel at any given moment, simply by changing the way we are breathing empowers us to live a better life!

Allow yourself the opportunity to get to know yourself better, to feel what it is like to really be you. We are all unique creations with something to share, and we owe it to ourselves to allow our true identities to surface. What I am sharing with you in this little book is a beginning to that discovery. By focusing on our breath coming in and going out, we allow our minds to take a break from all the other thoughts that constantly occupy our minds. As I stated before, we think thousands of thoughts a day, and the majority of those thoughts are the same ones that we thought yesterday and the day before. Trust yourself, your breath and the Universe, and know that we are all part of the whole. Tuning in and focusing on your breath, allows you to begin to make the connection to the real you, to your Source.

Our planet is in turmoil and humanity is going through a very difficult time. Our relationship to what is happening is all that we can really control. Be fully present with your breath, let go of everything else, feel the miracle of your body breathing, feel grateful for the miracle of your breath, feel gratitude for all you are and all you have. Even though it may not be everything you want, your life is a gift, and your breath is the doorway to that peace we are all longing for.

CHAPTER THREE

NOSTRIL BREATHING

Most instructions on breathing suggest that the inhalation is done through the nostrils and the exhalation is done through the mouth. However, during my Yoga teacher training, we were instructed to always breathe through the nostrils, both inhalations and exhalations.

Students have often asked me why they were told to exhale through their mouths and this is my response: My own personal understanding and belief is that when we are told to exhale through our mouths, we are told so because exhaling through the mouth guarantees more of a complete exhalation. This apparently is much easier for most people than to concentrate on exhaling completely.

Because the exhalation is so important, maybe it was felt that in order for someone to exhale more completely, it might be easier to do so through the mouth than the required concentration needed to exhale completely through the nostrils. If for some reason someone would have difficulty exhaling through their nostrils, then by all means, exhaling through the mouth would be necessary. However, I believe that we were provided nostrils for breathing and one must make every effort to learn to breathe through the nostrils and leave the mouth for speaking and eating.

Inhaling through our nostrils, holding the breath for just a moment, and then exhaling through our nostrils is the best and most beneficial way for us to breathe. Breathing into the abdomen, letting the breath expand the entire diaphragm and as the breath is exhaled, allowing the abdomen and diaphragm to slowly contract. If you've ever watched a baby sleeping, you've noticed the smooth easy rhythm of their breathing . . . this is how we are all meant to breath. We all breathed this way when we were babies, until we grew up and became caught up in all the craziness of the world. With a little practice, we can go back to that easy relaxed way of breathing, letting our Life Force fully enter our bodies and then slowly and completely letting it back out into the world.

CHAPTER FOUR

WE DON'T KNOW HOW TO BREATHE

We don't know how to breathe! That statement may sound ridiculous to say and to read, however it's true. Most of us breathe very shallowly using only the top portions of our lungs, and as a result we are not fully benefiting from each breath that comes in and out of our bodies. Our breath provides us with oxygen and simply put, **Our Breath Is Our Life Force**. We can survive without food, without water, however we can't live for more than a few moments without our breath.

My purpose in writing this little book is to help everyone learn how to breathe better. Those who have breathing issues or who, for whatever reason, have researched to find a better way to breathe have found a multitude of information available, both in books and on the internet. My intent is to provide some basic information in an easy to read format for those who wish to feel better, simply by breathing better. If you want to delve a little deeper, there are other more in-depth books available, as well as a multitude of information on the internet.

We all know that this is a very stressful time in which we live and my hope is that by bringing awareness to how important our breath is, and how easy it is to feel better by breathing better, others will be able to find the peace and relaxation that is the result of breathing with more focus and awareness. The simple fact is that if we pay attention to our breath, trying to bring in more and letting go more of this precious commodity, we will be able to find a sense of peace. When we are peaceful, we are better able to accept and cope with whatever life brings us.

Learning how to focus bringing the breath into the abdomen and learning how to exhale slowly and completely is the challenge. Letting go of our breath can be seen as a metaphor for life. Many of us have difficulty letting to—we tend to hold on to thoughts, material items, bad habits and sometimes even to people. Learning to exhale slowly and completely helps us to learn to let go. I like to look at the glass half empty/half full analogy from a different perspective. If the contents of the glass have become old, stagnant and spoiled, we need to empty out what's there in order to make room for fresh, clean and new. I like to think that when we exhale completely, we are eliminating all the old, which ultimately creates room for more fresh clean air to enter our bodies.

There seems to be a variety of medications available on the market today to help people who are having difficulty breathing. Why are we having trouble breathing? It's the most natural thing for these bodies to do, and yet there are very few people who are actually breathing well enough to derive the maximum benefit from each and every breath. My belief is that it has a lot to do with how stressed most of us are. You'll have to admit that there are so many things that we are bombarded with each and every day that cause us stress. Just watch the news at night and you will be sure to receive more unwanted bad news than you care to know about, however we still watch. I suggest you might try this little experiment—during the commercials, mute your television and close your eyes for a moment and take a few nice deep breathes. You might be surprised to find your attitude towards what you are seeing and hearing begins to change.

CHAPTER FIVE

EMPTYING THE LUNGS

We humans, for the most part, breathe very shallowly. When we breathe shallowly, we are inhaling limited amounts of air into our lungs, and then when we exhale we are not releasing that complete breath back out again. This means that we are retaining small amounts of air in our lungs. I don't know if this is a scientific fact or not, however the thought of accumulating stale air in my lungs because of not exhaling completely has helped me understand the importance of a complete exhalation, which has in turn helped me bring that awareness to my students. As a result of this shallow breathing, our lungs begin to lose the elasticity that they need to breathe deeply and completely.

With deep breaths we bring in more oxygen to nourish our bodies and minds, and when we exhale completely, we are releasing the toxins (carbon dioxide) back into the world to be recycled back into the oxygen that is breathed by all breathing organisms.

For this reason, it's in our best interest that we learn how to inhale deeply, and exhale completely thereby eliminating any air that may accumulate in our lungs as a result of shallow breathing. By exhaling completely, we will be able to provide the space in our lungs for the fresh clean air that our bodies and our minds need to thrive. And in learning how to exhale slowly and completely, it allows us to practice the art of letting go.

CHAPTER SIX

BREATHING TECHNIQUES

On the following pages I have described several breathing techniques which are easy to learn, and once you've practiced these techniques a few times, you'll begin to recognize how powerful they are. My suggestion is that you start slow, practicing each technique only a few times in the beginning, as you might feel a little lightheaded with the rush of oxygen and energy that you will be bringing into your body. You can practice these techniques anywhere at anytime and except for the Alternate Nostril Breathing, no one would ever know what you are doing.

There are available on the internet a video or two of some of these techniques, if you want a visual demonstration.

In addition to the benefits described for each technique, all of the techniques additionally offer the following benefits:

- An increase in the intake of oxygen helps to nourish the body and brain with the vital life force of breath.

- Any form of deep, mindful breathing can produce deep relaxation by clearing the mind and calming the body.

Breathing Technique One

ABDOMINAL BREATHING

a/k/a Diaphragmatic Breathing

This breathing technique is the most basic, and yet it might be the most difficult for some. The reason I say it might be the most difficult is because for many of us, stopping what we're doing, sitting down and beginning to take few deep breaths is a very difficult thing to do. However, once you have become comfortable with Abdominal Breathing, all the other techniques will be much easier to learn and accomplish.

In the beginning you might want to lie down. If you would rather sit in a chair, that's fine too—the most important thing is to try to keep your back straight. You may also want to place one of your hands on your belly and begin to bring your awareness to your breath coming in and going out. As you begin to focus on bringing your breath into your belly, you will feel your hand rise as you inhale and fall as you exhale.

With Abdominal Breathing, we want to bring the breath into the abdomen, so focus on this for a few moments, letting your hand rise and fall as you inhale and exhale into your belly. You can imagine your belly as a balloon, and as you inhale your breath is filling that balloon. As you exhale, the breath is leaving and you may imagine your belly as a deflating balloon, contracting and pulling inward. As I mentioned before, learning how to exhale slowly and completely is about letting go—something many of us have difficulty doing.

The most important outcome of practicing this breathing technique is to be able to bring awareness to your breath as it enters and leaves your body. If you have difficulty, just keep practicing and I guarantee that it won't take long before you will feel the rhythm of your breath coming in and going out, the gentle expanding and contracting of your belly.

As soon as your mind begins to focus on your breath, it is unable to think of anything else, and as a result the mind begins to relax and you'll notice that you are beginning to feel calm and peaceful. If you find your mind wandering and you're thinking about something other than your breath, gently bring your awareness back to your breath. In the beginning you might have to do this several times, however continue gently bringing your focus back to the breath, and eventually it will become easier and easier.

Benefits of Abdominal Breathing:

This is the most natural way to breathe. If you watch a baby breathing, you'll get an idea of this slow, deep and rhythmic way of breathing.

Abdominal/Diaphragmatic Breathing increases your awareness of your breathing patterns, balances your oxygen and carbon dioxide blood levels, normalizes the heart rate, and reduces muscle tension. It is the easiest way to begin to relax, improve your mood, reduce stress and promote overall health.

Breathing Technique Two

RELAXATION BREATHING

This breathing technique is very simple and I'm sure you'll have no problem mastering it almost immediately. Although you can do this breathing in any position, it's recommended that you sit with your back straight while you are learning.

The breath is inhaled through the nostrils to the count of four, then you'll hold the breath for the count of eight and finally release the breath through the nostrils to the count of eight.

- Sit comfortably with a straight back.
- **Inhale** through the nostrils to a count of **four.**
- **Hold** the breath to the count of **eight.**
- **Exhale** through the nostrils to a count of **eight.**
- **Repeat**

This breathing technique is a natural tranquilizer for the entire nervous system and increases in power the more often you practice. In the beginning, for the first few weeks, you might begin practicing twice a day, doing no more than three or four breaths at a time. As you become more comfortable with the technique, you might extend it to eight breaths. There is no such thing as doing this too much.

If you are trying these breathing techniques for the first time, you might find yourself feeling a little lightheaded when you first begin to breathe this way, however there is no reason for alarm—it will pass. Again, it's just the rush of oxygen and energy that you are bringing into your body that is causing this feeling. Stop for the time being, and continue when the lightheadedness passes.

Once you have become comfortable with Relaxation Breathing, you will most likely want it to become part of your life. As the name implies, you can use it whenever you feel upset, allowing you to calm yourself before reacting. This way of breathing will relax you anytime you feel anxious, frustrated or feel any kind of internal tension. It's also very helpful if you are having trouble falling asleep. Everyone of any age will benefit from practicing Relaxation Breathing.

Benefits of Relaxation Breathing:

Relaxation Breathing allows your entire system to come back into balance by deepening your breathing, reducing stress hormones, slowing down your heart rate and blood pressure, and relaxing your muscles and your mind.

In addition to its calming physical effects, research shows that allowing your body and mind to relax in this way also increases energy and focus, helps to combat illness, relieves aches and pains, heightens problem-solving abilities, and boosts motivation and productivity.

Breathing Technique Three

THREE PART BREATHING

Our breath is our primary source of energy. Three part breathing allows us the greatest absorption of oxygen into the body as well as expelling the toxic air (carbon dioxide)

This technique expands on the Abdominal Breathing that you have already learned.

- As you inhale, feel the breath being pulled down into your belly. Now, let it begin to rise up into your chest and then up into your throat (the clavicle area). Allow the breath to completely fill the body slowly from the bottom, to the middle and up to the top.
- Hold the breath for just a moment and now begin to release the breath first from the throat (clavicle area), descending down into the chest and finally out of the belly, pulling your belly flat expelling as much air as you are able.
- Repeat the inhalation and exhalation as described above.

This way of breathing enables you to experience a smooth flowing of the breath as it comes in from the bottom of the belly, rising up filling the body, and then releasing it back down and out.

I suggest trying to visualize in your mind an ocean wave washing onto shore. As you inhale, imagine bringing the wave (your breath) up onto the shore, and as you exhale, let your breath push the wave back out to sea.

Practice this breathing technique as long as you are comfortable. Once you find your own unique rhythm, you'll begin to feel relaxed and your breathing will naturally begin to settle down back into the abdomen.

Benefits of Three Part Breathing:

Relaxation through focused mindful breathing brings your entire system back into balance deepening your breathing, reducing stress hormones, slowing down your heart rate and blood pressure, and relaxing your muscles.

In addition to its calming physical effects, research shows that the relaxation which results from focused mindful breathing also increases energy and focus, combats illness, relieves aches and pains, and heightens problem-solving abilities. Best of all, everyone is capable of learning to breathe properly and thereby benefits in the process.

Breathing Technique Four

ALTERNATE NOSTRIL BREATHING

Alternate Nostril Breathing is a breathing technique which alternates inhaling and exhaling from one nostril to the next. Breathing naturally alternates from one nostril to the next about every two hours, however we are not aware of this occurring as the change happens on its own. Generally when someone suffers from congestion in one nostril, it stops the natural alternating air flow from left to right nostril. This can lead to problems.

Please read this entire section completely before beginning to practice Alternate Nostril Breathing.

- Sit in a chair or on the floor being sure to keep the spine as straight as possible.
- Hold your right hand up and turn your pointer and middle finger down, curling them into your palm. This leaves the thumb, ring and pinky fingers available.
- Your thumb will be used to close your right nostril and your ring and pinky fingers to close your left nostril, alternating from one side to the other.

- **Begin** by covering your right nostril with your thumb and **inhaling** through the **left** nostril filling the entire abdominal cavity to the count of 4.

- Using your ring and pinky fingers, **close** off the **left** nostril and with thumb still on the right nostril, **hold** the breath for 4-16 counts (depending on experience level).

- Then **release** the thumb from the **right** nostril and slowly **exhale** to the count of 4-8 (depending on experience level).

- **Inhale** into the **right** nostril, close both nostrils and **hold** for 4-16 counts before releasing the ring and pinky fingers and **exhaling** through the **left** nostril.

- **Inhale** into the **left** nostril, **hold** and **repeat exhale** on the **right,** and then **inhale** on the **right** side, **holding** and **exhaling** through the **left.**

Additional Important Points to Know:

- When you first begin this practice, inhale for 4 counts, hold for 4 counts, and exhale for 4 counts.

- The general rule is always inhale to the count of 4, holding the breath up to the count of 16, and exhaling up to the count of 8. As you become comfortable with the process of alternating the nostrils, you can increase the count to a maximum of 4-16-8. Inhaling for a count of 4, holding for a count of 16 and exhaling for a count of 8. During my Yoga teacher training, I was taught that the maximum count of the exhale should be twice the amount of the inhale, and the hold to be four times the inhale, thus 4-16-8. Work up to this count slowly and don't try the maximum count until you are comfortable . . . . there's no hurry. Just relax and enjoy.

- Three cycles minimum should be performed by always beginning with the left nostril inhalation.

- In the beginning practice this breathing for 5 minutes at a time and increase up to 10 minutes.

- It is important to stay relaxed and calm through this breathing. At first it may seem unnatural but eventually it will become more relaxing and soothing.

- You may experience a little runny nose as you practice this technique, as several of my students have reported. I believe that this is because there's a mild congestion in your nasal passages that begins to work loose as you practice Alternate Nostril Breathing.

Cautions:

- This breathing should *not* be practiced if you have a cold or a sinus infection that would cause total blockage of one or both nasal passages.
- This breathing technique should *not* be practiced too vigorously or too excessively.
- If you are pregnant, please check with your doctor before practicing any breathing exercises that require any sort of breath retention.

Benefits of Alternate Nostril Breathing:

- Alternate Nostril Breathing can produce deep relaxation by clearing the mind and calming the body, and is a great preparation for meditation, as well as any type of creative work.
- The holding of the breath between inhales and exhales helps to regulate and direct the flow of breath in the body, helping to maximize benefits and the flow of our Life Force.
- Alternate Nostril Breathing helps to balance the left and right hemispheres of the brain (linear thinking and creative thinking).

- Alleviates headaches and calms anxiety and tense mental states.

- Alternate Nostril Breathing helps to regulate the heating and cooling cycles of the body.

WHEN TO USE THESE BREATHING TECHNIQUES

In the morning take a few deep Abdominal Breaths allowing yourself to feel a sense of gratitude for the miracle of your breath. As you inhale, you may want to open your arms wide stretching open the chest so that you can begin to expand your lungs as well as opening your heart.

Anytime you find yourself *beginning* to feel fearful, anxious, angry, or developing a sense of being uncomfortable for any reason, this is when you might want to practice Abdominal Breathing and then work into Three Part Breathing. Continue focusing on your breath until you begin to feel yourself relaxing and feeling a sense of calmness. After you've used these techniques a few times, you will begin to recognize that it doesn't require much effort, or much time, to bring yourself back to your center, the place where you are relaxed and peaceful.

More intense feelings of stress will call for Relaxation Breathing and Alternate Nostril Breathing. These techniques require more concentration and need the mind more. Because you are engaging the mind more, it begins to relax quicker as you bring your focus to your Life Force coming in and going out, counting and breathing.

Learning and practicing these techniques will reward you with being able to control your breathing, your mind, your feelings and your actions.

CHAPTER SEVEN

FINAL THOUGHTS

In writing *Breathing Better—Feeling Better*, I've tried to create a format that is easy to read and understand so that everyone has the opportunity to learn how important their breath is to their life. My hope is that you'll use your breath to begin to slow down so that you are able to relax into that peaceful place that is your true nature.

In the beginning, it will take several times a day to practice in order for you to feel comfortable with each technique. When you are practicing, it's best that you wear comfortable clothing that will allow your abdomen to expand and contract easily. Choose the particular technique you want to practice, find a comfortable quiet place to sit down, and begin. The hardest part is to actually sit down and begin to focus on your breath! Sometimes the easiest things are the hardest . . . . maybe because they *are* so easy.

After you have become comfortable with this new way of breathing, you can use these techniques in any situation. Once I was standing in line at the airport and beginning to feel very anxious. The line was long and moving very slowly, and the people in line with me were beginning to show signs of agitation and restlessness. As soon as I brought awareness to my breath, coming in and going out, I almost immediately began to feel relaxed and accepting of the situation. The coolest part was that I made eye contact with a woman who was smiling and just emitting such a sense of calm compared to most of the other people in line . . . . we smiled at each other. Here was a situation where dozens of people found themselves in a very uncomfortable position and were becoming more and more agitated as time went on. While on the other hand, there were at least two of us (hopefully more) that weren't allowing the circumstances that we found ourselves in to get the better of us, and were managing to maintain a sense of calm acceptance. This is a perfect example of what I'm talking about . . . . it's not what is happening to us, it's about how we are *feeling* about what is happening.

We only have the power to change how we feel. The world is what it is. Being able to create and nurture this feeling of acceptance, especially when we are in an uncomfortable situation is the challenge. It's only a challenge when you're first beginning, because after you've become familiar with the techniques, and have proven to yourself that they work, you'll find yourself automatically bringing awareness to your breath, pulling back from the situation and going to that peaceful place where your breath takes you. Even though you are still here in the world of craziness, you aren't allowing the outside craziness to make *you* crazy. You will have learned how to function in the world from a more peaceful center, which not only is beneficial for you; it will ultimately have positive effects on everyone around you and your environment. Just imagine if we all became more relaxed and peaceful!

When we begin to breathe better, making a deeper connection with our breath, we begin to become more accepting of what is. Being more aware allows us the ability to better manage our lives. Stress is wishing that the present moment is different than it is. If you want something different, you have the opportunity to change the future, however being able to accept this moment as it is, whatever it may be is peace!

Try to bring your awareness to the breath as you inhale in the Life Force, feeling it enter your body feeding each and every cell. And, as you exhale slowly and completely, bring your awareness to releasing and letting go. If this way of breathing is practiced, and allowed to become second nature to you, it will bring you to a place of gratitude and acceptance, which is peace, our true nature.

On a deeper level, my understanding is that Planet Earth has actually shifted on its axis and we are all feeling the effects of that shift. Many believe that Mother Earth is actually speaking to us by way of floods, tsunamis, earthquakes, and global warming—we're beginning to get a sense that she isn't happy.

Recently I heard that the rumblings and shakings are actually from Mother Earth being pregnant, giving birth to a higher consciousness, a new awareness. There is a shift that has occurred that we are all feeling, despite our not being able to identify or even understand what is happening.

The world is in turmoil, we humans are going through a very difficult time, individually and collectively. It's important that we remember who we are and live life from that center. Even though there have been tough times, and maybe more tough times are to come, just know that deep inside, away from all the constant ups and downs of your life, there is a place of peace—your true nature. You only need to be willing to Breathe Better so that you can Feel Better.

After reading this, I'm hoping that you'll begin to realize that there is a way for you to take back a little control for how you feel. There's something that you can do so that the craziness that is permeating our world will not have an adverse effect on you. Everyone has to do this for his or herself, it's an individual activity, and we can't sit back and expect others to make the changes we want to see happen. If we want change, a better world, it begins with each of us taking responsibility for our own selves, trying to become the best that we can be. I believe it's our own individual contribution to the world, our payback for all that we have been blessed with. We must all begin to slow down and relax the constant movement of our minds. Let go of all those thoughts so that we can hear that Still Small Voice, Our True Self, our Power Source—the Mother Ship! ☺

Prayer is communicating with God. Mindful breathing is communicating with our own Selves. They require the same dedication to practice in order to make the strength of those connections stronger and stronger. If we all concentrated on our own inner lights to guide us and let other people tend to their own light, the result would be that we would all begin to see and feel more fully how we are all in this together. We are like one big team—"The Humans".

What I'm hoping to accomplish by writing this little book, is to make available to those that are looking for a way to feel better, some things that I've learned along the way that have helped me become more peaceful, more accepting, and more grateful for each and every breath that enters and leaves my body. I have tried to provide information about how important breathing properly is and sharing some techniques to accomplish this. I've also shared some of my thoughts, and some of my own realizations along the way. So, what I'm hoping to do is make available for those that are looking, a way that they can begin to help themselves feel better, which leads to those around them feeling better, and ultimately to help the world (Mother Earth) feel better.

All I'm suggesting is that if you are really serious about wanting to feel better, you'll try to sit down for a few minutes and bring awareness to your breath. If we all become more peaceful, with less fear and anger, think about how much better this world could be. Just imagine all the children on Mother Earth playing happily together. We all have the ability to feel better, to be more peaceful, and one of the ways to feel this peace comes with learning to better use and appreciate our breath, the Universal Life Force that flows through each and every living organism that we share this planet with. If we want a better world, we must all begin to focus on becoming the best that we can be. Learning to breathe better, allowing our bodies and minds to become more relaxed, peaceful and accepting, I believe is the beginning of creating the world we all would like to see.

Namaste'

Hopi Mindfulness

There is a river flowing now very fast.

It is so great and so swift, that there are those who will be afraid.

They will feel they are being torn apart and will suffer greatly.

Know that the river has its destination.

The elders say we must let go of the shore, push off into the middle of the river.

Keep our eyes open and our heads above the water.

And they say to see who is there with you and celebrate.

At this time in history, we are to take nothing personally, least of all ourselves, for the moment that we do, our spiritual growth and journey come to a halt.

The time of the lone wolf is over.

Gather yourselves.

Banish the word struggle from your vocabulary.

All that we do now must be done in a sacred manner and in celebration.

We are the ones we have been waiting for.

~ Message from the Hopi Elders ~